Heart Health Breakthrough

Proven Strategies for a Vibrant and Resilient Heart"

By AURORA GLORY

Table of Content

Introduction: Understanding Heart Health

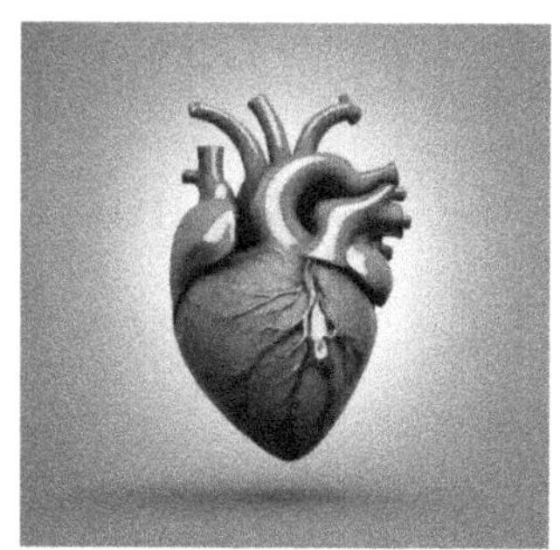

Importance of Heart Health

Heart health is a crucial aspect of overall well-being and longevity. The heart, a muscular organ roughly the size of a fist, is responsible for pumping blood throughout the body. This vital function delivers oxygen and nutrients to tissues and removes waste products. Because of its central role in sustaining life, maintaining a healthy heart is fundamental to preserving one's quality of life and preventing serious health issues.

Heart disease remains the leading cause of death globally. According to the World Health Organization (WHO), cardiovascular diseases account for nearly 32% of all global deaths. This statistic underscores the importance of prioritizing heart health to prevent such conditions and their associated complications.

Several factors contribute to the critical nature of heart health. First, the heart's performance directly impacts other bodily functions. Efficient circulation ensures that organs, muscles, and tissues receive adequate nutrients and oxygen, which is essential for their optimal functioning. Poor heart health can lead to fatigue, reduced physical performance, and even organ dysfunction.

Moreover, heart disease can have a profound effect on one's quality of life. Conditions like coronary artery disease, heart attacks, and heart failure can limit physical activity, reduce the ability to perform daily tasks, and affect mental health. For instance, individuals with heart disease often experience increased levels of anxiety and depression, further exacerbating their overall health.

Maintaining heart health is also economically beneficial. Treating heart disease and its complications involves significant medical costs, including hospitalizations, medications, and long-term care. By investing in heart health through preventive measures and lifestyle changes, individuals can potentially reduce these expenses and alleviate the burden on healthcare systems.

Overview of Heart Disease Risks

Understanding the risks associated with heart disease is essential for effective prevention and management. Several factors contribute to the development of cardiovascular conditions, and they can be broadly categorized into modifiable and non-modifiable risks.

1. Modifiable Risk Factors

- Unhealthy Diet: Diets high in saturated fats, trans fats, cholesterol, and sodium can lead to the development of atherosclerosis, where plaque builds up in the arteries, narrowing them and restricting blood flow. Consuming excessive amounts of processed foods and sugary beverages can also contribute to obesity, a significant risk factor for heart disease.

- Physical Inactivity: Regular physical activity strengthens the heart muscle, improves circulation, and helps manage weight. A sedentary lifestyle, on the other hand, is linked to a higher risk of cardiovascular diseases. Lack of exercise can contribute to obesity, high blood pressure, and elevated cholesterol levels.

- Smoking: Tobacco smoke contains harmful chemicals that damage blood vessels and promote the buildup of plaque in the arteries. Smoking significantly increases the risk of heart disease and stroke. Quitting smoking can substantially reduce this risk and improve overall heart health.

- Excessive Alcohol Consumption: While moderate alcohol consumption may have some protective effects on heart health, excessive drinking can lead to high blood pressure, heart disease, and liver damage. It's important to consume alcohol in moderation to mitigate these risks.

- Chronic Stress: Persistent stress can lead to unhealthy behaviors such as poor eating habits, smoking, and excessive alcohol consumption. Stress also affects the cardiovascular system by increasing blood pressure and promoting inflammation, which can contribute to heart disease.

2. Non-Modifiable Risk Factors
- Age: The risk of heart disease increases with age. As people get older, their blood vessels naturally become stiffer and less elastic, which can contribute to higher blood pressure and increased risk of cardiovascular events.

- Gender: Men generally have a higher risk of heart disease at a younger age compared to women. However, the risk for women increases and can surpass that of men after menopause due to hormonal changes that affect heart health.

- Genetics and Family History: A family history of heart disease can increase an individual's risk of developing similar conditions. Genetic predispositions can influence factors such as cholesterol levels, blood pressure, and the overall function of the heart.

- Ethnicity: Certain ethnic groups are at a higher risk for heart disease. For example, individuals of African American, Hispanic, and South Asian descent often have higher rates of hypertension and diabetes, both of which are risk factors for heart disease.

Understanding heart health and the risks associated with heart disease is the first step toward prevention and management. By addressing modifiable risk factors such as diet, physical activity, and lifestyle choices, individuals can take proactive measures to protect their heart health. Additionally, being aware of non-modifiable risk factors can help in making informed decisions and seeking appropriate medical guidance. Ultimately, prioritizing heart health not only enhances overall well-being but also reduces the risk of serious cardiovascular conditions and improves quality of life.

The Anatomy of a Healthy Heart

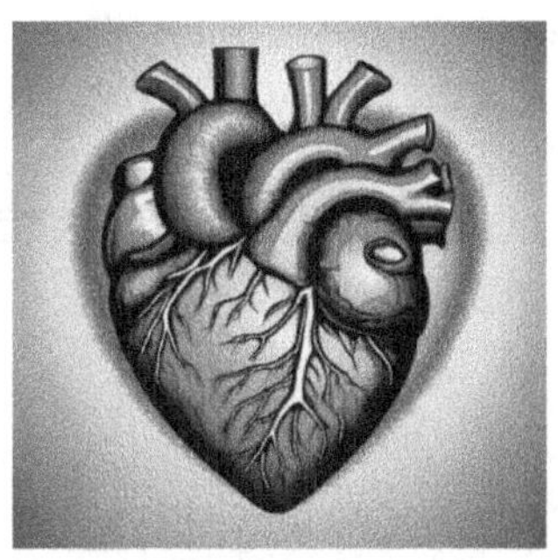

How the Heart Works

The heart is an extraordinary organ with a sophisticated structure that enables it to perform its critical role of pumping blood throughout the body. Understanding the anatomy of the heart and how it functions is fundamental to grasping how to maintain heart health and prevent cardiovascular diseases.

1. Structure of the Heart

The heart is a muscular organ located in the chest cavity, slightly to the left of the midline. It is roughly the size of a fist and consists of four chambers: two atria (upper chambers) and two ventricles (lower chambers). The heart's structure is designed to efficiently circulate blood through two distinct pathways: the pulmonary circulation and the systemic circulation.

- Atria: The right atrium receives deoxygenated blood from the body via the superior and inferior vena cava. The left atrium receives oxygenated blood from the lungs via the pulmonary veins. These chambers act as receiving areas that prepare blood for the next phase of circulation.

- Ventricles: The right ventricle pumps deoxygenated blood into the pulmonary artery, which carries it to the lungs for oxygenation. The left ventricle, which is the strongest of the four chambers, pumps oxygenated blood into the aorta, the largest artery in the body. The aorta then distributes blood to the rest of the body.

2. Valves of the Heart

The heart contains four main valves that ensure blood flows in the correct direction and prevents backflow:

- Tricuspid Valve: Located between the right atrium and right ventricle, it prevents blood from flowing backward into the atrium when the ventricle contracts.

- Pulmonary Valve: Positioned between the right ventricle and the pulmonary artery, it prevents blood from flowing back into the ventricle after it has been ejected into the artery.

- Mitral Valve: Located between the left atrium and left ventricle, it prevents blood from flowing backward into the atrium during ventricular contraction.

- Aortic Valve: Found between the left ventricle and the aorta, it prevents blood from flowing back into the ventricle after it has been pumped into the aorta.

3. The Cardiac Cycle

The heart's function is regulated through the cardiac cycle, which consists of two main phases: systole and diastole.

- Systole: This is the phase when the heart muscle contracts. During systole, the ventricles contract to pump blood out of the heart. The right ventricle sends blood to the lungs, while the left ventricle sends blood to the rest of the body.

- Diastole: This is the phase when the heart muscle relaxes. During diastole, the heart chambers fill with blood. The atria fill with blood from the body and lungs, and this blood then moves into the ventricles as they relax.

4. Electrical Conduction System

The heart's ability to beat in a coordinated manner is controlled by its electrical conduction system. This system generates and transmits electrical impulses that regulate the heart's rhythm and ensure efficient blood pumping:

- Sinoatrial (SA) Node: Often referred to as the heart's natural pacemaker, the SA node is located in the right atrium. It initiates electrical impulses that cause the atria to contract and push blood into the ventricles.

- Atrioventrikulær (AV) Node: Located at the junction between the atria and ventricles, the AV node receives impulses from the SA node and delays them slightly to allow the ventricles to fill with blood before contracting.

- Bundle of His and Purkinje Fibers: The electrical impulse travels from the AV node through the Bundle of His and into the Purkinje fibers, which spread the impulse throughout the ventricles, causing them to contract and pump blood out of the heart.

Key Factors for Maintaining Heart Health

Maintaining heart health involves understanding and addressing several key factors that impact the overall function and condition of the heart. By focusing on these areas, individuals can promote cardiovascular health and reduce the risk of heart disease.

1. Nutrition

A balanced and heart-healthy diet is essential for maintaining cardiovascular health. Key dietary recommendations include:

- Healthy Fats: Incorporate sources of unsaturated fats, such as avocados, nuts, seeds, and olive oil. These fats can help reduce LDL (bad) cholesterol levels and increase HDL (good) cholesterol levels.

- Whole Grains: Choose whole grains like oats, brown rice, and whole wheat bread over refined grains. Whole grains are high in fiber, which can help lower cholesterol levels and improve heart health.

- Fruits and Vegetables: A diet rich in fruits and vegetables provides essential vitamins, minerals, and antioxidants. These nutrients support heart health by reducing inflammation and improving blood vessel function.

- Lean Proteins: Opt for lean protein sources such as fish, poultry, beans, and legumes. Fish, especially fatty fish like salmon, is high in omega-3 fatty acids, which have been shown to reduce the risk of heart disease.

- Sodium and Sugar: Limit the intake of sodium and added sugars. Excessive sodium can raise blood pressure, while high sugar consumption is linked to obesity and diabetes, both of which are risk factors for heart disease.

2. Physical Activity

Regular exercise is crucial for maintaining a healthy heart. Physical activity helps:

- Strengthen the Heart Muscle: Regular cardiovascular exercise, such as walking, running, or swimming, improves the heart's efficiency and endurance.

- Manage Weight: Exercise helps regulate body weight, which is important for controlling risk factors like high blood pressure and high cholesterol.

- Reduce Stress: Physical activity stimulates the release of endorphins, which can help manage stress and improve mood, contributing to overall heart health.

- Improve Circulation: Exercise enhances blood flow and helps keep blood vessels flexible and healthy, reducing the risk of atherosclerosis.

3. Stress Management

Chronic stress can have a negative impact on heart health by increasing blood pressure and contributing to unhealthy behaviors. Effective stress management techniques include:

- Relaxation Techniques: Practices such as deep breathing, meditation, and progressive muscle relaxation can help reduce stress and lower blood pressure.

- Physical Activity: Regular exercise is not only beneficial for physical health but also serves as a natural stress reliever.

- Healthy Hobbies: Engaging in activities that bring joy and relaxation, such as reading, gardening, or spending time with loved ones, can help alleviate stress.

4. Regular Check-Ups

Routine medical check-ups are essential for monitoring heart health and detecting potential issues early. Key aspects to monitor include:

- Blood Pressure: Regularly check blood pressure to ensure it remains within a healthy range. High blood pressure can damage blood vessels and increase the risk of heart disease.

- Cholesterol Levels: Monitor cholesterol levels to ensure a healthy balance of LDL and HDL cholesterol. High LDL levels can lead to plaque buildup in the arteries.

- Blood Sugar Levels: Keep track of blood sugar levels to prevent or manage diabetes, which is a significant risk factor for heart disease.

5. Avoiding Harmful Habits

Certain habits can negatively affect heart health. Avoiding these behaviors is crucial for maintaining cardiovascular well-being:

- Smoking: Smoking is a major risk factor for heart disease. It damages blood vessels, increases blood pressure, and contributes to plaque buildup. Quitting smoking is one of the most significant steps one can take to improve heart health.

- Excessive Alcohol Consumption: Limit alcohol intake to moderate levels. Excessive drinking can lead to high blood pressure, heart disease, and liver damage.

6. Healthy Weight Management

Maintaining a healthy weight is vital for heart health. Excess weight, particularly around the abdomen, is associated with increased risk of cardiovascular conditions. Strategies for weight management include:

- Balanced Diet: Follow a nutritious diet that supports weight control without compromising on essential nutrients.

- Regular Exercise: Incorporate physical activity into daily routines to burn calories and support healthy weight maintenance.

- Portion Control: Pay attention to portion sizes to avoid overeating and unnecessary calorie consumption.

Nutrition for a Strong Heart

Essential Nutrients for Heart Health

A well-balanced diet plays a crucial role in maintaining heart health and preventing cardiovascular disease. The heart requires a variety of nutrients to function optimally, and certain nutrients have been shown to specifically support cardiovascular health. Understanding these essential nutrients and how they contribute to heart health can help individuals make informed dietary choices that promote a strong, healthy heart.

1. Omega-3 Fatty Acids

Omega-3 fatty acids are a type of polyunsaturated fat that have been extensively studied for their heart-protective effects. They are found in high concentrations in fatty fish such as salmon, mackerel, and sardines. Omega-3s are known for their ability to:

- Reduce Inflammation: Omega-3 fatty acids have anti-inflammatory properties that help lower inflammation in the body, which is a key factor in the development of heart disease.

- Lower Blood Pressure: Regular consumption of omega-3s can help reduce blood pressure levels, which in turn lowers the risk of heart disease.

- Improve Cholesterol Levels: Omega-3s help increase HDL (good) cholesterol levels while decreasing triglycerides, which can reduce the risk of plaque buildup in the arteries.

2. Fiber

Dietary fiber, particularly soluble fiber, is beneficial for heart health. Soluble fiber can be found in foods such as oats, barley, beans, and certain fruits and vegetables. Fiber contributes to heart health in several ways:

- Lower Cholesterol Levels: Soluble fiber binds to cholesterol in the digestive tract, helping to reduce LDL (bad) cholesterol levels and prevent it from being absorbed into the bloodstream.

- Regulate Blood Sugar Levels: Fiber helps slow the absorption of sugar, which can help manage blood sugar levels and reduce the risk of developing diabetes—a risk factor for heart disease.

- Promote Healthy Weight: High-fiber foods are often low in calories and help increase satiety, which can aid in weight management and reduce obesity-related heart risks.

3. Antioxidants

Antioxidants are compounds that help protect the body's cells from oxidative stress and damage. They are abundant in fruits, vegetables, nuts, and seeds. Key antioxidants beneficial for heart health include:

- Vitamin C: Found in citrus fruits, berries, and leafy greens, vitamin C helps protect the heart by reducing inflammation and oxidative damage.

- Vitamin E: Present in nuts, seeds, and green leafy vegetables, vitamin E helps prevent oxidative damage to cells and supports overall cardiovascular health.

- Polyphenols: These compounds are found in foods such as berries, dark chocolate, and green tea. Polyphenols have anti-inflammatory and antioxidant properties that support heart health.

4. Potassium

Potassium is a mineral essential for maintaining healthy blood pressure levels. It helps balance the effects of sodium and relaxes blood vessel walls, contributing to lower blood pressure. Key sources of potassium include:

- Fruits: Bananas, oranges, and avocados are rich in potassium.
- Vegetables: Sweet potatoes, spinach, and tomatoes provide significant amounts of potassium.
- Legumes: Beans and lentils are also good sources of this mineral.

5. Magnesium

Magnesium plays a vital role in maintaining normal heart rhythm and supporting overall cardiovascular health. It helps regulate blood pressure and supports muscle function, including the heart muscle. Magnesium can be found in:

- Nuts and Seeds: Almonds, sunflower seeds, and pumpkin seeds are high in magnesium.
- Whole Grains: Brown rice, quinoa, and whole wheat products provide magnesium.
- Leafy Greens: Spinach and kale are excellent sources of magnesium.

Heart-Healthy Diet Plans

Adopting a heart-healthy diet involves incorporating a variety of foods that support cardiovascular health and making lifestyle changes to improve overall well-being. Here are some key dietary patterns and plans that promote heart health:

1. The Mediterranean Diet

The Mediterranean diet is renowned for its heart-health benefits and emphasizes:

- Healthy Fats: Focus on sources of unsaturated fats, such as olive oil, nuts, and avocados. These fats are beneficial for lowering LDL cholesterol and reducing inflammation.

- Lean Proteins: Incorporate fish, poultry, and legumes as primary protein sources. Fatty fish rich in omega-3s are particularly encouraged.

- Fruits and Vegetables: A wide variety of fruits and vegetables are included to provide essential vitamins, minerals, and antioxidants.

- Whole Grains: Opt for whole grains such as whole wheat bread, brown rice, and quinoa instead of refined grains.

- Herbs and Spices: Use herbs and spices like garlic, basil, and oregano to add flavor and reduce the need for added salt.

2. The DASH Diet

The Dietary Approaches to Stop Hypertension (DASH) diet is designed to lower blood pressure and improve heart health. Its key components include:

- Low Sodium: Reduce sodium intake to help manage blood pressure levels. This involves cutting back on processed and packaged foods high in salt.

- High in Fruits and Vegetables: Emphasize fresh fruits and vegetables for their potassium, fiber, and antioxidant content.

- Whole Grains: Choose whole grains such as oats, barley, and whole wheat products.

- Lean Proteins: Incorporate lean meats, poultry, and fish, along with plant-based protein sources like beans and legumes.

- Low-Fat Dairy: Opt for low-fat or fat-free dairy products to reduce saturated fat intake.

3. Plant-Based Diet

A plant-based diet focuses on foods derived from plants and can provide numerous benefits for heart health. This diet includes:

- Fruits and Vegetables: High consumption of a variety of fruits and vegetables ensures intake of essential nutrients and antioxidants.

- Legumes: Beans, lentils, and chickpeas are rich sources of protein, fiber, and essential minerals.

- Nuts and Seeds: Include a variety of nuts and seeds for their healthy fats and nutrients.

- Whole Grains: Incorporate whole grains like quinoa, barley, and brown rice.

- Minimized Animal Products: Limit or eliminate the intake of meat and dairy products, focusing instead on plant-based alternatives.

Foods to Avoid

Certain foods can negatively impact heart health and increase the risk of cardiovascular disease. To maintain a healthy heart, it is important to limit or avoid the following:

1. Saturated and Trans Fats

Saturated and trans fats can raise LDL cholesterol levels and contribute to the development of atherosclerosis. Foods high in these fats include:

- **Red Meat:** Fatty cuts of beef, pork, and lamb can be high in saturated fat.
- Processed Meats: Sausages, hot dogs, and bacon often contain high levels of saturated fats and preservatives.
- Fried Foods: Foods fried in oils high in trans fats, such as certain fast foods and baked goods, should be avoided.

2. Excessive Sodium

High sodium intake is linked to elevated blood pressure, which is a significant risk factor for heart disease. Foods to limit include:

- Processed and Packaged Foods: Many canned soups, frozen meals, and snacks contain high levels of sodium.
- Salty Snacks: Potato chips, pretzels, and other salty snacks contribute to excessive sodium intake.

3. Added Sugars

Excessive consumption of added sugars can lead to weight gain, obesity, and increased risk of type 2 diabetes. Foods and beverages high in added sugars include:

- Sugary Drinks: Soda, energy drinks, and sweetened teas can contribute to high sugar intake.
- Candy and Sweets: Candies, pastries, and sugary desserts can add large amounts of added sugars to the diet.

4. Refined Carbohydrates

Refined carbohydrates can cause rapid spikes in blood sugar levels and contribute to weight gain. Foods to avoid include:

- White Bread: Made from refined flour, which lacks fiber and essential nutrients.
- Pastries and Baked Goods: Often made with refined flour and high in added sugars and unhealthy fats.

The Role of Exercise in Heart Health

Exercise is a cornerstone of cardiovascular health. Regular physical activity not only strengthens the heart but also enhances overall well-being. By understanding how exercise benefits the cardiovascular system, individuals can adopt effective exercise strategies to support heart health, create balanced routines, and integrate movement into daily life.

Effective Exercises for Cardiovascular Fitness

Cardiovascular exercises, often referred to as aerobic exercises, are crucial for improving heart health. These activities increase the heart rate, enhance blood circulation, and boost cardiovascular endurance. Here are several effective exercises for cardiovascular fitness:

1. Running and Jogging

Running and jogging are fundamental cardiovascular exercises that elevate heart rate and promote cardiovascular health. These activities offer numerous benefits:

- Cardiovascular Endurance: Running and jogging improve the efficiency of the heart and lungs, enhancing overall cardiovascular endurance.
- Caloric Expenditure: These exercises burn a significant number of calories, which can aid in weight management and reduce the risk of obesity-related heart disease.
- Mental Health Benefits: Running and jogging also release endorphins, which can improve mood and reduce stress.

2. Cycling

Cycling is an excellent form of low-impact cardiovascular exercise that can be done indoors or outdoors. Its benefits include:

- Joint-Friendly: The low-impact nature of cycling makes it suitable for individuals with joint issues or those recovering from injury.
- Varied Intensity: Cycling can be adjusted for different intensity levels, from leisurely rides to high-intensity interval training (HIIT).
- Improved Cardiovascular Health: Regular cycling improves heart function and endurance, supports weight management, and can lower blood pressure.

3. Swimming

Swimming provides a comprehensive workout for cardiovascular fitness and is particularly beneficial due to its low-impact nature. Key benefits of swimming include:

- Full-Body Exercise: Swimming engages multiple muscle groups, offering a full-body workout that enhances cardiovascular and muscular fitness.
- Buoyancy: The buoyancy of water reduces stress on joints, making it an ideal exercise for individuals with arthritis or other joint issues.
- Enhanced Lung Capacity: Regular swimming improves respiratory function and lung capacity.

4. Walking

Walking is one of the most accessible and versatile forms of cardiovascular exercise. Its benefits are:

- Low Impact: Walking is gentle on the joints, making it suitable for individuals of all fitness levels.
- Accessibility: Walking requires no special equipment and can be done almost anywhere, from neighborhood streets to indoor tracks.

- Health Benefits: Regular walking improves cardiovascular health, helps manage weight, and can reduce the risk of chronic diseases.

5. High-Intensity Interval Training (HIIT)

HIIT involves alternating periods of intense activity with periods of rest or lower-intensity exercise. This approach offers:

- Efficiency: HIIT workouts are time-efficient and can provide significant cardiovascular benefits in a shorter duration.
- Increased Metabolism: HIIT can boost metabolism and continue to burn calories after the workout has ended.
- Improved Fitness: This method enhances cardiovascular endurance and can improve overall fitness levels.

Creating a Balanced Exercise Routine

A balanced exercise routine incorporates various types of physical activities to ensure comprehensive fitness and promote heart health. Here are key components for creating a balanced routine:

1. Cardiovascular Exercise

Cardiovascular or aerobic exercises are essential for improving heart health. To achieve optimal benefits:

- Frequency: Aim for at least 150 minutes of moderate-intensity aerobic exercise or 75 minutes of vigorous-intensity exercise per week, as recommended by the American Heart Association.
- Variety: Incorporate a mix of activities such as walking, running, cycling, and swimming to keep workouts engaging and address different aspects of cardiovascular fitness.

2. Strength Training

Strength training is crucial for building muscle mass, supporting metabolic health, and enhancing overall fitness. To include strength training:

- Frequency: Perform strength training exercises at least two days per week.
- Muscle Groups: Target major muscle groups, including the chest, back, legs, and arms, using exercises such as squats, lunges, push-ups, and rows.
- Resistance Levels: Use free weights, resistance bands, or body weight to provide adequate resistance and challenge muscles.

3. Flexibility and Mobility

Flexibility and mobility exercises support joint health and prevent injuries. Incorporate:

- Static Stretching: Perform static stretches after exercise to improve flexibility and reduce muscle stiffness.
- Dynamic Stretching: Include dynamic stretches as part of your warm-up routine to prepare the body for physical activity.

4. Balance and Core Stability

Balance and core stability exercises enhance overall fitness and support functional movement:

- Balance Exercises: Engage in activities that improve balance, such as standing on one leg or using a balance board.
- Core Exercises: Strengthen the core with exercises like planks, Russian twists, and bicycle crunches to support stability and prevent injury.

5. Rest and Recovery

Rest and recovery are essential for preventing overtraining and allowing the body to repair and strengthen:

- Rest Days: Schedule at least one or two rest days per week to give muscles time to recover.
- Active Recovery: Engage in low-intensity activities like gentle walking or stretching on rest days to promote circulation and aid recovery.

Incorporating Movement into Daily Life

Integrating movement into daily routines helps maintain an active lifestyle and supports heart health, even with a busy schedule. Consider these strategies:

1. Active Commuting

Incorporate physical activity into your commute:

- Walking or Biking: Walk or bike for short trips instead of driving. If using public transportation, consider getting off one stop early and walking the rest of the way.
- Parking Further Away: Park further from your destination to increase walking distance.

2. Workplace Activity

Stay active throughout the workday:

- Stand and Move: Use a standing desk or take short walking breaks to reduce sedentary time.
- Desk Exercises: Perform simple exercises or stretches at your desk to stay active.

3. Family and Social Activities
Engage in physical activities with family and friends:

- Family Activities: Participate in active family outings such as hiking, biking, or playing sports.
- Social Fitness: Join group fitness classes or sports teams to combine social interaction with physical activity.

4. Home Workouts
Create opportunities for exercise at home:
- Home Exercise Routine: Develop a home workout routine using body weight exercises, resistance bands, or free weights.
- Active Chores: Engage in household chores like vacuuming or gardening, which can contribute to daily physical activity.

5. Leisure Activities
Choose hobbies that involve physical activity:
- Active Hobbies: Pursue hobbies such as dancing, gardening, or playing sports that keep you moving and active.
- Outdoor Activities: Spend time outdoors engaging in activities like hiking, kayaking, or playing recreational sports.

6. Set Realistic Goals

Establish achievable fitness goals to stay motivated:

- SMART Goals: Set Specific, Measurable, Achievable, Relevant, and Time-bound goals to track progress and maintain focus.
- Gradual Progress: Start with small, manageable goals and gradually increase intensity or duration as fitness improves.

7. Overcoming Barriers

Address common barriers to maintaining an active lifestyle:

- Time Constraints: Schedule exercise sessions into your day or break workouts into shorter segments to fit into a busy schedule.
- Lack of Motivation: Find activities you enjoy, set rewarding milestones, and exercise with a friend or group for added motivation.
- Physical Limitations: Adapt exercises to accommodate physical limitations or injuries, and consult a fitness professional for guidance.

The Psychological Benefits of Exercise

Exercise offers significant psychological benefits that complement physical health improvements:

1. Stress Reduction

Physical activity helps manage and reduce stress:

- Endorphin Release: Exercise promotes the release of endorphins, which are natural mood enhancers that reduce stress and anxiety.
- Mental Clarity: Engaging in regular exercise can improve mental clarity and provide a break from daily stressors.

2. Enhanced Cognitive Function

Regular exercise supports brain health and cognitive function:

- Improved Blood Flow: Exercise increases blood flow to the brain, which supports cognitive function and memory.
- Neurogenesis: Physical activity promotes neurogenesis, the creation of new neurons, which is essential for cognitive health.

3. Better Sleep

Exercise can improve sleep quality and duration:

- Sleep Regulation: Regular physical activity helps regulate sleep patterns and promotes deeper, more restorative sleep.
- Reduced Insomnia: Engaging in exercise can help alleviate symptoms of insomnia and improve overall sleep quality.

4. Boosted Self-Esteem

Achieving fitness goals and experiencing physical improvements can enhance self-esteem:

- Sense of Achievement: Meeting exercise goals and witnessing physical progress can provide a sense of accomplishment and boost confidence.
- Positive Body Image: Regular exercise can lead to improvements in body composition and self-perception, enhancing body image.

Managing Stress for a Healthy Heart

Stress is a pervasive aspect of modern life, impacting not only mental well-being but also physical health, particularly cardiovascular health. Understanding how stress affects the heart and employing effective stress management techniques are essential for maintaining a healthy heart. This comprehensive exploration delves into the impact of stress on heart health, techniques for stress reduction, and mindfulness and relaxation practices that contribute to overall well-being.

Impact of Stress on Heart Health

Stress affects cardiovascular health through several physiological and behavioral mechanisms. Chronic stress can have detrimental effects on the heart and increase the risk of developing cardiovascular diseases.

1. Physiological Effects of Stress

- Increased Heart Rate and Blood Pressure: During periods of stress, the body's "fight-or-flight" response is activated, leading to increased heart rate and elevated blood pressure. Chronic activation of this response can strain the cardiovascular system and contribute to hypertension.

- Inflammatory Response: Stress triggers the release of stress hormones such as cortisol and adrenaline. Prolonged exposure to these hormones can lead to increased inflammation in the body, which is a risk factor for atherosclerosis (the buildup of plaques in the arteries) and heart disease.
- Blood Clotting: Stress has been linked to changes in blood clotting mechanisms. Increased levels of stress hormones can lead to a higher risk of blood clots, which may contribute to heart attacks or strokes.
- Immune System Impact: Chronic stress can weaken the immune system, making the body more susceptible to infections and potentially exacerbating cardiovascular conditions.

2. Behavioral Effects of Stress
- Unhealthy Coping Mechanisms: Individuals under stress may engage in unhealthy behaviors such as smoking, excessive alcohol consumption, or overeating, all of which negatively impact heart health.
- Sedentary Lifestyle: Stress can lead to decreased physical activity as individuals may lack motivation or energy to exercise. A sedentary lifestyle is associated with a higher risk of cardiovascular disease.
- Poor Sleep: Stress often disrupts sleep patterns, leading to poor sleep quality and insufficient rest. Chronic sleep deprivation can contribute to hypertension, obesity, and other cardiovascular risk factors.

3. Long-Term Cardiovascular Risks

Chronic stress is associated with several long-term cardiovascular risks:

- Hypertension: Prolonged stress can lead to persistent high blood pressure, a major risk factor for heart disease and stroke.
- Coronary Artery Disease: Stress-induced inflammation and blood clotting can contribute to the development of coronary artery disease, which involves the narrowing of the coronary arteries due to plaque buildup.
- Heart Attack: Chronic stress is linked to an increased risk of heart attacks. The combined effects of stress hormones, inflammation, and unhealthy behaviors can heighten the likelihood of experiencing a myocardial infarction.

Techniques for Stress Reduction

Managing stress effectively is crucial for maintaining heart health. Employing a variety of stress reduction techniques can help mitigate the adverse effects of stress and promote overall well-being.

1. Physical Activity

Exercise is one of the most effective stress management techniques and offers numerous cardiovascular benefits:

- Aerobic Exercise: Engaging in aerobic exercises such as walking, running, cycling, or swimming helps reduce stress by promoting the release of endorphins, which are natural mood enhancers.
- Strength Training: Incorporating strength training exercises into your routine can also help manage stress and improve cardiovascular health.
- Consistency: Regular physical activity is key to maintaining stress reduction benefits. Aim for at least 150 minutes of moderate-intensity aerobic exercise per week, combined with strength training exercises on two or more days per week.

2. Healthy Diet

A balanced diet can play a significant role in stress management and heart health:

- Nutrient-Rich Foods: Consume a diet rich in fruits, vegetables, whole grains, lean proteins, and healthy fats. These foods provide essential nutrients that support overall health and help manage stress.
- Limit Caffeine and Sugar: Reduce intake of caffeine and sugary foods, as these can exacerbate stress and negatively affect heart health.
- Hydration: Staying hydrated is important for overall health and can help manage stress levels.

3. Social Support

Building and maintaining strong social connections can help manage stress:

- Social Interactions: Engage in social activities and maintain relationships with friends and family. Positive social interactions can provide emotional support and reduce stress.
- Support Groups: Consider joining support groups or participating in community activities to build a network of individuals who can offer support and encouragement.

4. Time Management

Effective time management can help reduce stress by improving organization and reducing feelings of overwhelm:

- Prioritize Tasks: Identify and prioritize tasks to focus on what is most important. Break tasks into manageable steps to make them less overwhelming.
- Set Realistic Goals: Set achievable goals and avoid overcommitting. Allocate time for breaks and relaxation to prevent burnout.

5. Relaxation Techniques

Incorporating relaxation techniques into your daily routine can help reduce stress:

- Deep Breathing: Practice deep breathing exercises to calm the nervous system and reduce stress. Techniques such as diaphragmatic breathing or the 4-7-8 method can be effective.
- Progressive Muscle Relaxation: This technique involves tensing and then relaxing different muscle groups to release physical tension and promote relaxation.
- Visualization: Use guided imagery or visualization techniques to create calming mental images and reduce stress.

Mindfulness and Relaxation Practices

Mindfulness and relaxation practices are powerful tools for managing stress and supporting cardiovascular health. These practices promote relaxation, improve emotional regulation, and enhance overall well-being.

1. Mindfulness Meditation

Mindfulness meditation involves focusing on the present moment and observing thoughts and sensations without judgment. Benefits include:

- Stress Reduction: Mindfulness meditation helps reduce stress by promoting relaxation and enhancing self-awareness.
- Improved Emotional Regulation: Regular mindfulness practice can improve emotional regulation and reduce symptoms of anxiety and depression.
- Enhanced Cardiovascular Health: Mindfulness has been linked to lower blood pressure and improved heart health.

2. Yoga

Yoga combines physical postures, breathing exercises, and meditation to promote relaxation and stress reduction:

- Physical Benefits: Yoga improves flexibility, strength, and balance, contributing to overall physical health.
- Mental Benefits: Yoga encourages relaxation and mental clarity, helping to reduce stress and anxiety.
- Cardiovascular Health: Regular yoga practice can lower blood pressure and improve heart rate variability, contributing to better cardiovascular health.

3. Tai Chi

Tai Chi is a gentle martial art that involves slow, deliberate movements and deep breathing:

- Stress Relief: Tai Chi promotes relaxation and reduces stress through its slow, meditative movements.
- Improved Balance and Flexibility: Regular practice improves balance, flexibility, and overall physical health.
- Cardiovascular Benefits: Tai Chi has been shown to improve cardiovascular health by lowering blood pressure and enhancing heart rate variability.

4. Guided Imagery

Guided imagery involves using mental images to promote relaxation and reduce stress:

- Relaxation Response: Visualization techniques can help elicit the relaxation response, reducing stress and promoting a sense of calm.
- Stress Reduction: Guided imagery can be used to create calming mental scenarios that help alleviate stress and anxiety.
- Enhancing Well-Being: Regular use of guided imagery can improve overall emotional well-being and support cardiovascular health.

5. Mindfulness-Based Stress Reduction (MBSR)

MBSR is an evidence-based program that combines mindfulness meditation with body awareness techniques:

- Structured Program: MBSR typically involves an eight-week program with weekly classes and daily mindfulness practices.
- Health Benefits: Research shows that MBSR can reduce stress, improve emotional regulation, and enhance overall well-being.
- Cardiovascular Health: MBSR has been associated with improvements in blood pressure and cardiovascular risk factors.

6. Progressive Muscle Relaxation (PMR)

PMR involves tensing and then relaxing different muscle groups to reduce physical tension and stress:

- Physical Relaxation: PMR helps release muscle tension and promote physical relaxation.
- Stress Reduction: By focusing on the process of tensing and relaxing muscles, PMR can reduce overall stress levels.
- Improved Sleep: PMR can also improve sleep quality by promoting relaxation and reducing symptoms of insomnia.

The Connection Between Sleep and Heart Health

Sleep is a vital component of overall health, influencing various physiological processes and playing a crucial role in maintaining cardiovascular well-being. Understanding the connection between sleep and heart health is essential for optimizing both. This comprehensive examination explores the importance of quality sleep, provides tips for improving sleep quality, and discusses the impact of sleep disorders on heart health.

Importance of Quality Sleep

Quality sleep is fundamental for maintaining cardiovascular health and overall well-being. During sleep, the body undergoes various restorative processes that are crucial for heart health and metabolic balance.

1. Cardiovascular Repair and Restoration

- Blood Pressure Regulation: Sleep helps regulate blood pressure. During deep sleep stages, blood pressure typically decreases, providing a resting period for the cardiovascular system. Chronic sleep deprivation can lead to sustained high blood pressure, increasing the risk of hypertension and heart disease.

- Heart Rate Variability: Quality sleep promotes healthy heart rate variability (HRV), an indicator of the autonomic nervous system's ability to respond to stress and maintain cardiovascular health. Lower HRV is associated with an increased risk of cardiovascular problems.
- Endothelial Function: Sleep supports the health of the endothelium, the thin layer of cells lining blood vessels. Adequate sleep helps maintain endothelial function, which is crucial for proper blood flow and preventing atherosclerosis.

2. Metabolic Health and Weight Management

- Insulin Sensitivity: Quality sleep is linked to improved insulin sensitivity, which helps regulate blood sugar levels. Poor sleep can lead to insulin resistance, a precursor to type 2 diabetes, which is a significant risk factor for cardiovascular disease.
- Appetite Regulation: Sleep influences hormones that regulate appetite, such as leptin and ghrelin. Lack of sleep can disrupt these hormones, leading to increased appetite and poor dietary choices, which can contribute to obesity and cardiovascular risk.
- Weight Management: Adequate sleep supports healthy weight management. Obesity is a major risk factor for heart disease, and poor sleep quality can contribute to weight gain and obesity.

3. Inflammation and Immune Function

- Inflammatory Markers: Quality sleep helps regulate inflammatory responses in the body. Chronic sleep deprivation is associated with elevated levels of inflammatory markers, which can contribute to the development of cardiovascular diseases.
- Immune System Support: Sleep is essential for a well-functioning immune system. A robust immune system helps protect against infections and supports cardiovascular health by reducing inflammation and promoting overall health.

4. Cognitive and Emotional Health

- Cognitive Function: Sleep supports cognitive function, including memory, attention, and problem-solving skills. Poor sleep can impair cognitive function and contribute to stress and anxiety, which can negatively affect cardiovascular health.
- Emotional Regulation: Quality sleep plays a role in emotional regulation and mental health. Chronic sleep deprivation can lead to mood disturbances and increased stress, which can have adverse effects on heart health.

Tips for Improving Sleep Quality

Improving sleep quality is essential for maintaining cardiovascular health and overall well-being. Implementing effective sleep strategies can enhance sleep quality and promote better heart health.

1. Establish a Consistent Sleep Schedule

- Regular Sleep Routine: Aim to go to bed and wake up at the same time every day, even on weekends. Consistency helps regulate the body's internal clock and improves sleep quality.
- Bedtime Rituals: Develop a relaxing bedtime routine, such as reading a book or taking a warm bath, to signal to the body that it's time to wind down.

2. Create a Sleep-Friendly Environment

- Comfortable Sleep Environment: Ensure your sleep environment is comfortable and conducive to rest. This includes a comfortable mattress and pillows, as well as a cool, dark, and quiet room.
- Limit Light Exposure: Reduce exposure to artificial light in the evening, especially blue light from screens. Blue light can interfere with melatonin production, a hormone that regulates sleep.

3. Practice Relaxation Techniques

- Deep Breathing: Practice deep breathing exercises to promote relaxation and reduce stress before bedtime.
- Progressive Muscle Relaxation: Engage in progressive muscle relaxation to release physical tension and prepare the body for sleep.

- Mindfulness Meditation: Incorporate mindfulness meditation to calm the mind and reduce anxiety, helping to improve sleep quality.

4. Limit Stimulants and Heavy Meals
- Caffeine and Nicotine: Avoid consuming caffeine and nicotine in the hours leading up to bedtime. Both substances can interfere with the ability to fall asleep and negatively affect sleep quality.
- Heavy Meals: Refrain from eating large or heavy meals close to bedtime, as they can cause discomfort and disrupt sleep.

5. Exercise Regularly
- Physical Activity: Engage in regular physical activity to promote better sleep. Exercise helps regulate sleep patterns and reduces symptoms of insomnia.
- Timing: Avoid vigorous exercise too close to bedtime, as it can be stimulating and interfere with the ability to fall asleep.

6. Manage Stress
- Stress Reduction: Implement stress management techniques to reduce anxiety and promote relaxation. Chronic stress can negatively impact sleep quality and overall health.
- Time Management: Practice effective time management to reduce stress and avoid feelings of overwhelm that can interfere with sleep.

7. Monitor Sleep Patterns

- Sleep Tracking: Use a sleep tracker or journal to monitor sleep patterns and identify factors that may be affecting sleep quality.
- Adjustments: Make necessary adjustments to sleep habits based on tracking data to improve sleep quality and overall well-being.

Sleep Disorders and Heart Health

Sleep disorders can have a significant impact on heart health, and addressing these conditions is crucial for maintaining cardiovascular well-being.

1. Obstructive Sleep Apnea (OSA)

- Description: OSA is a common sleep disorder characterized by repeated episodes of blocked airflow during sleep. These episodes can lead to intermittent drops in oxygen levels and fragmented sleep.
- Cardiovascular Risks: OSA is associated with an increased risk of hypertension, coronary artery disease, heart failure, and stroke. The repeated interruptions in breathing and oxygen levels can strain the cardiovascular system.

- Management: Treatment options for OSA include continuous positive airway pressure (CPAP) therapy, lifestyle modifications, and, in some cases, surgical interventions.

2. Insomnia

- Description: Insomnia is characterized by difficulty falling asleep or staying asleep, leading to poor sleep quality and daytime impairment.
- Cardiovascular Risks: Chronic insomnia is linked to an increased risk of hypertension, cardiovascular disease, and impaired glucose metabolism. The associated stress and anxiety can contribute to cardiovascular problems.
- Management: Treatment for insomnia may include cognitive-behavioral therapy for insomnia (CBT-I), relaxation techniques, and lifestyle changes to improve sleep hygiene.

3. Restless Legs Syndrome (RLS)

- Description: RLS is a condition characterized by uncomfortable sensations in the legs and an urge to move them, often leading to difficulty falling asleep.
- Cardiovascular Risks: While RLS itself is not directly linked to cardiovascular disease, the sleep disturbances caused by the condition can contribute to increased stress and cardiovascular risk.

- Management: Treatment options for RLS include lifestyle changes, medications, and addressing underlying conditions that may contribute to the symptoms.

4. Narcolepsy

- Description: Narcolepsy is a chronic sleep disorder characterized by excessive daytime sleepiness and sudden sleep attacks. It can also involve abnormal sleep patterns, such as rapid eye movement (REM) sleep occurring immediately upon falling asleep.
- Cardiovascular Risks: The impact of narcolepsy on cardiovascular health is not fully understood, but disrupted sleep patterns and excessive daytime sleepiness may contribute to increased cardiovascular risk.
- Management: Treatment for narcolepsy may include medications to manage symptoms and lifestyle adjustments to improve sleep quality and daytime alertness.

5. Circadian Rhythm Disorders

- Description: Circadian rhythm disorders involve disruptions in the body's internal clock, affecting sleep-wake patterns and overall sleep quality.

- Cardiovascular Risks: Disrupted circadian rhythms are associated with an increased risk of hypertension, metabolic disorders, and cardiovascular disease. Shift work and irregular sleep patterns can contribute to these risks.

- Management: Strategies for managing circadian rhythm disorders include maintaining a consistent sleep schedule, exposure to natural light during the day, and addressing factors that disrupt circadian rhythms.

Preventive Measures and Regular Check-Ups

Preventive measures and regular check-ups are essential components of maintaining heart health and preventing cardiovascular diseases. Engaging in proactive health practices and monitoring key health indicators can significantly reduce the risk of heart-related conditions and enhance overall well-being. This comprehensive guide delves into the importance of regular heart screenings, understanding blood pressure and cholesterol levels, and the role of preventive medications in cardiovascular health.

Importance of Regular Heart Screenings

Regular heart screenings are crucial for early detection and management of cardiovascular issues. These screenings help identify risk factors and existing conditions before they escalate into more severe health problems.

1. Early Detection of Heart Disease

- Identifying Risk Factors: Regular screenings can help detect risk factors such as high blood pressure, elevated cholesterol levels, and abnormal heart rhythms. Early identification allows for timely intervention and lifestyle modifications to reduce the risk of developing heart disease.

- Detecting Asymptomatic Conditions: Many cardiovascular conditions, such as atherosclerosis or heart disease, may not present obvious symptoms until they reach an advanced stage. Regular screenings can identify these conditions before symptoms develop, allowing for earlier and more effective treatment.

2. Monitoring Existing Conditions

- Managing Chronic Conditions: For individuals with known cardiovascular conditions, regular check-ups are essential for monitoring disease progression and adjusting treatment plans as needed. This includes conditions such as hypertension, coronary artery disease, and heart failure.
- Assessing Treatment Efficacy: Regular screenings help evaluate the effectiveness of prescribed treatments and medications. Adjustments can be made based on these assessments to optimize heart health and prevent complications.

3. Risk Stratification and Prevention

- Personalized Risk Assessment: Heart screenings provide a comprehensive assessment of cardiovascular risk factors, enabling healthcare providers to develop personalized prevention strategies. This includes recommendations for lifestyle changes, dietary adjustments, and preventive medications.

- Guiding Preventive Measures: Regular check-ups help guide preventive measures such as smoking cessation, weight management, and physical activity. Addressing these risk factors can significantly reduce the likelihood of developing heart disease.

Understanding Blood Pressure and Cholesterol Levels

Blood pressure and cholesterol levels are critical indicators of cardiovascular health. Understanding these parameters is essential for managing heart health and preventing cardiovascular disease.

1. Blood Pressure

- Normal Blood Pressure Levels: Blood pressure is measured in millimeters of mercury (mm Hg) and consists of two readings: systolic (the pressure when the heart beats) and diastolic (the pressure when the heart rests between beats). Normal blood pressure is typically below 120/80 mm Hg.

- Hypertension: High blood pressure, or hypertension, is defined as a reading of 130/80 mm Hg or higher. Hypertension is a major risk factor for heart disease, stroke, and kidney damage. It can often be asymptomatic, making regular monitoring crucial.

- Managing Blood Pressure: Maintaining a healthy blood pressure involves lifestyle modifications such as a balanced diet, regular exercise, reducing salt intake, and managing stress. In some cases, medications may be prescribed to help control blood pressure levels.

2. Cholesterol Levels

- Types of Cholesterol: Cholesterol is a fatty substance present in the blood. Key types include low-density lipoprotein (LDL) cholesterol, often referred to as "bad" cholesterol, and high-density lipoprotein (HDL) cholesterol, known as "good" cholesterol. Elevated LDL levels and low HDL levels are associated with an increased risk of heart disease.

- Cholesterol Levels and Cardiovascular Risk: A total cholesterol level below 200 mg/dL is generally considered desirable. LDL levels below 100 mg/dL are optimal, while HDL levels above 60 mg/dL are protective. Elevated total cholesterol or LDL levels can contribute to plaque buildup in the arteries, leading to atherosclerosis and cardiovascular disease.

- Managing Cholesterol: Lifestyle changes such as adopting a heart-healthy diet, increasing physical activity, and avoiding smoking can help manage cholesterol levels. Medications, such as statins, may be prescribed to lower LDL cholesterol and reduce cardiovascular risk.

Preventive Medications and Their Role

Preventive medications play a vital role in reducing the risk of cardiovascular diseases, particularly for individuals with specific risk factors or pre-existing conditions.

1. Statins

- Function: Statins are a class of medications used to lower LDL cholesterol levels in the blood. By reducing LDL cholesterol, statins help prevent the buildup of plaque in the arteries, reducing the risk of heart attacks and strokes.
- Indications: Statins are commonly prescribed to individuals with elevated LDL cholesterol levels, a history of cardiovascular disease, or multiple risk factors for heart disease. They are also used in primary prevention for individuals with a high risk of developing cardiovascular disease.

2. Aspirin

- Function: Aspirin is an antiplatelet medication that helps prevent blood clots by inhibiting platelet aggregation. It is often used to reduce the risk of heart attacks and strokes, particularly in individuals with a history of cardiovascular events.
- Indications: Low-dose aspirin may be recommended for individuals with a history of heart disease, stroke, or certain risk factors such as diabetes or a family history of cardiovascular disease.

However, its use in primary prevention (for individuals without a history of cardiovascular events) is more nuanced and should be based on individual risk assessments.

3. ACE Inhibitors and ARBs

- Function: Angiotensin-converting enzyme (ACE) inhibitors and angiotensin II receptor blockers (ARBs) are medications that help lower blood pressure and reduce the workload on the heart. They work by relaxing blood vessels and improving blood flow.
- Indications: These medications are commonly prescribed for individuals with hypertension, heart failure, or chronic kidney disease. They can also help reduce the risk of cardiovascular events in individuals with certain risk factors.

4. Beta-Blockers

- Function: Beta-blockers are medications that reduce heart rate and lower blood pressure by blocking the effects of adrenaline. They help decrease the heart's workload and improve symptoms in individuals with heart conditions.
- Indications: Beta-blockers are prescribed for individuals with heart failure, coronary artery disease, or a history of heart attacks. They can also be used to manage certain arrhythmias and reduce the risk of cardiovascular events.

5. Diuretics

- Function: Diuretics, also known as "water pills," help reduce fluid buildup in the body by increasing urine output. This can help lower blood pressure and reduce symptoms of heart failure.
- Indications: Diuretics are commonly prescribed for individuals with hypertension, heart failure, or fluid retention. They are often used in combination with other medications to manage cardiovascular conditions.

6. Anticoagulants

- Function: Anticoagulants, such as warfarin or direct oral anticoagulants (DOACs), help prevent blood clot formation by inhibiting the clotting process. They are used to reduce the risk of strokes and other thrombotic events.
- Indications: Anticoagulants are prescribed for individuals with atrial fibrillation, deep vein thrombosis, or a history of blood clots. They are used to prevent clot-related complications and reduce cardiovascular risk.

7. Lifestyle Modifications

- Role in Prevention: While not medications, lifestyle modifications are a critical aspect of preventive cardiovascular care. Changes such as adopting a heart-healthy diet, engaging in regular physical activity, quitting smoking, and managing stress can significantly reduce cardiovascular risk and complement the effects of preventive medications.

Lifestyle Changes for Long-Term Heart Health

Lifestyle changes are pivotal in maintaining long-term heart health and preventing cardiovascular diseases. Adopting healthy habits can significantly reduce the risk of heart-related conditions and improve overall well-being. This guide delves into three critical areas for enhancing heart health: smoking cessation, moderation of alcohol consumption, and maintaining a healthy weight. Each section provides comprehensive strategies and insights to support lasting heart health improvements.

Smoking Cessation Strategies

Smoking is a major risk factor for cardiovascular diseases, including coronary artery disease, stroke, and peripheral artery disease. The harmful chemicals in tobacco smoke damage blood vessels, increase blood pressure, and promote the buildup of plaque in the arteries. Quitting smoking is one of the most impactful changes an individual can make for heart health. Here are effective strategies to help with smoking cessation:

1. Understanding the Impact of Smoking

- Cardiovascular Damage: Smoking accelerates the development of atherosclerosis by promoting the oxidation of LDL cholesterol and causing inflammation in the arterial walls. It also increases the risk of blood clots by making blood platelets more sticky.

- Heart Disease Risks: Smokers are more likely to develop coronary artery disease and experience heart attacks compared to non-smokers. Quitting smoking reduces the risk of these conditions and improves overall cardiovascular health.

2. Developing a Quit Plan

- Set a Quit Date: Choose a specific date to stop smoking and prepare for it by gathering support and resources. Marking this date on the calendar can serve as a motivational milestone.

- Identify Triggers: Recognize situations, emotions, or activities that trigger the urge to smoke. Developing strategies to cope with these triggers, such as finding alternative activities or practicing stress-relief techniques, can be beneficial.

- Seek Support: Engage in support groups, counseling, or smoking cessation programs. Professional help can provide guidance, encouragement, and accountability throughout the quitting process.

3. Using Nicotine Replacement Therapy (NRT)

- Types of NRT: Nicotine replacement products, such as nicotine patches, gum, lozenges, and inhalers, can help manage withdrawal symptoms and reduce cravings. These products provide a controlled dose of nicotine without the harmful chemicals found in cigarettes.
- Effectiveness: NRT has been shown to double the chances of quitting smoking compared to trying to quit without assistance. Combining NRT with behavioral therapy can further enhance the likelihood of success.

4. Prescription Medications

- Varenicline (Chantix): Varenicline reduces nicotine cravings and withdrawal symptoms by affecting brain receptors involved in nicotine addiction. It can also decrease the pleasure derived from smoking.
- Bupropion (Zyban): Bupropion is an antidepressant that can help with smoking cessation by reducing withdrawal symptoms and cravings. It may be prescribed to individuals who have not succeeded with other methods.

5. Behavioral Strategies

- Cognitive-Behavioral Therapy (CBT): CBT helps individuals identify and change negative thought patterns and behaviors associated with smoking. It can be effective in managing cravings and developing coping strategies.

- Mindfulness and Stress Management: Practicing mindfulness and relaxation techniques can help manage stress and reduce the urge to smoke. Techniques such as deep breathing, meditation, and yoga can be beneficial.

6. Lifestyle Adjustments

- Healthy Substitutes: Replace smoking with healthier habits, such as physical activity, hobbies, or social interactions. Engaging in activities that provide satisfaction and distract from cravings can aid in quitting.

- Avoiding Triggers: Stay away from environments or situations where smoking is prevalent. If certain social settings or stressors trigger the urge to smoke, develop alternative coping mechanisms or avoid these triggers when possible.

Moderation of Alcohol Consumption

Excessive alcohol consumption is linked to various health issues, including hypertension, heart disease, and liver damage. Moderating alcohol intake can significantly benefit heart health and overall wellness. Here are strategies for managing alcohol consumption:

1. Understanding the Effects of Alcohol

- Cardiovascular Risks: Heavy alcohol consumption can lead to high blood pressure, irregular heartbeats, and cardiomyopathy (a condition where the heart muscle weakens). It also increases the risk of developing heart disease and stroke.
- Moderation Benefits: Reducing alcohol intake lowers the risk of developing cardiovascular issues, improves liver function, and enhances overall health. Moderation can also lead to better sleep quality and weight management.

2. Setting Limits and Goals

- Daily and Weekly Limits: The American Heart Association recommends limiting alcohol consumption to no more than one drink per day for women and two drinks per day for men. One drink is typically defined as 12 ounces of beer, 5 ounces of wine, or 1.5 ounces of distilled spirits.
- Personal Goals: Set realistic and specific goals for reducing or eliminating alcohol consumption. This could include designating alcohol-free days, gradually reducing intake, or seeking support for complete abstinence if needed.

3. Choosing Healthier Alternatives

- Low-Alcohol Options: Opt for beverages with lower alcohol content or consider non-alcoholic alternatives. Many brands offer non-alcoholic beers and mocktails that can provide similar flavors without the alcohol.
- Hydration: Drink plenty of water and non-alcoholic beverages to stay hydrated and reduce the likelihood of excessive alcohol consumption. Drinking water between alcoholic beverages can also help moderate intake.

4. Social Strategies

- Communicate Your Goals: Inform friends and family about your intention to moderate alcohol consumption. Their support and understanding can help you stay accountable and reduce social pressures to drink.
- Find Alternative Activities: Engage in social activities that do not revolve around alcohol. Exploring new hobbies, attending events, or participating in group activities can provide enjoyable experiences without the need for alcohol.

5. Seeking Support

- Counseling and Therapy: If alcohol consumption becomes a significant issue, consider seeking professional help. Counseling or therapy can provide support, strategies, and tools for managing alcohol use and addressing any underlying issues.
- Support Groups: Join support groups or organizations dedicated to alcohol moderation or abstinence. Sharing experiences and receiving encouragement from others with similar goals can be beneficial.

Maintaining a Healthy Weight

Obesity and being overweight are major risk factors for heart disease, hypertension, and diabetes. Maintaining a healthy weight through balanced nutrition and regular physical activity is essential for long-term heart health. Here are strategies for achieving and sustaining a healthy weight:

1. Understanding the Impact of Weight on Heart Health

- Cardiovascular Risks: Excess body weight can contribute to high blood pressure, high cholesterol levels, and insulin resistance. It also places additional strain on the heart and can lead to the development of heart disease.

- Benefits of Weight Management: Achieving and maintaining a healthy weight can reduce the risk of cardiovascular disease, improve blood pressure and cholesterol levels, and enhance overall health and quality of life.

2. Adopting a Balanced Diet

- Healthy Eating Habits: Focus on a diet rich in fruits, vegetables, whole grains, lean proteins, and healthy fats. Avoid processed foods, high-sugar snacks, and excessive saturated and trans fats.
- Portion Control: Pay attention to portion sizes and avoid overeating. Using smaller plates, measuring servings, and practicing mindful eating can help manage calorie intake.
- Meal Planning: Plan meals in advance to ensure they are balanced and nutritious. Preparing meals at home allows for better control over ingredients and portion sizes.

3. Engaging in Regular Physical Activity

- Types of Exercise: Incorporate a mix of cardiovascular exercises (such as walking, jogging, or swimming), strength training (such as weight lifting or resistance exercises), and flexibility activities (such as yoga or stretching).
- Exercise Recommendations: Aim for at least 150 minutes of moderate-intensity aerobic activity or 75 minutes of vigorous-

intensity activity per week, along with muscle-strengthening activities on two or more days a week.

- Consistency: Make physical activity a regular part of your routine. Find activities you enjoy and set realistic goals to stay motivated and maintain an active lifestyle.

4. Behavioral Strategies

- Goal Setting: Set specific, achievable goals for weight management. This could include targets for weight loss, physical activity, or dietary changes. Tracking progress and celebrating milestones can provide motivation.
- Mindful Eating: Practice mindful eating by paying attention to hunger and fullness cues. Avoid eating out of boredom, stress, or emotional triggers, and focus on enjoying meals and snacks.

5. Monitoring and Support

- Regular Monitoring: Track weight, body measurements, and other health indicators to monitor progress and make necessary adjustments to your weight management plan.
- Seek Professional Guidance: Consult with healthcare providers or registered dietitians for personalized advice and support. They can help develop a tailored weight management plan and address any specific health concerns.

6. Addressing Emotional and Psychological Factors

- Emotional Eating: Identify and address emotional eating triggers, such as stress, boredom, or anxiety. Developing healthier coping mechanisms, such as engaging in hobbies or seeking support, can help manage emotional eating.
- Support Networks: Surround yourself with supportive friends, family, and communities that encourage healthy habits and provide motivation. Support groups or counseling can also be beneficial for addressing emotional and psychological aspects of weight management.

Managing Existing Heart Conditions

Managing existing heart conditions is crucial for improving quality of life and preventing the progression of cardiovascular diseases. Effective management involves understanding common heart conditions, exploring medication and treatment options, and employing coping strategies to handle chronic heart disease. This comprehensive guide provides an in-depth look into these aspects to help individuals manage their heart health proactively.

Common Heart Conditions and Their Management

Several heart conditions are prevalent and require specific management strategies to control symptoms, prevent complications, and improve overall heart health.

1. Hypertension (High Blood Pressure)

- Overview: Hypertension is a condition where the blood pressure in the arteries is persistently elevated. It is a major risk factor for heart disease, stroke, and kidney damage. Normal blood pressure is generally considered to be below 120/80 mm Hg, while hypertension is defined as blood pressure readings of 130/80 mm Hg or higher.
- Management: Managing hypertension involves lifestyle changes and medications:

- Lifestyle Changes: Adopting a heart-healthy diet (such as the DASH diet), reducing sodium intake, maintaining a healthy weight, and engaging in regular physical activity can help lower blood pressure. Limiting alcohol consumption and quitting smoking are also beneficial.

- Medications: Common medications include diuretics, ACE inhibitors, angiotensin II receptor blockers (ARBs), beta-blockers, and calcium channel blockers. These medications work by reducing blood pressure and preventing related complications.

2. Coronary Artery Disease (CAD)

- Overview: CAD occurs when the coronary arteries, which supply blood to the heart muscle, become narrowed or blocked due to atherosclerosis. This can lead to chest pain (angina) and heart attacks.

- Management: Managing CAD focuses on relieving symptoms and preventing progression:

- Lifestyle Modifications: Adopting a heart-healthy diet, engaging in regular exercise, managing stress, and quitting smoking are key. Weight management and controlling cholesterol levels are also important.

- Medications: Medications such as statins, aspirin, beta-blockers, and ACE inhibitors are used to manage CAD. Statins help lower LDL cholesterol, while aspirin reduces the risk of blood clots.

- Procedures: In some cases, procedures like angioplasty and stenting or coronary artery bypass grafting (CABG) may be necessary to restore blood flow to the heart.

3. Heart Failure

- Overview: Heart failure is a condition in which the heart is unable to pump blood effectively, leading to fluid buildup in the lungs and other parts of the body. It can be caused by various conditions, including CAD, hypertension, and cardiomyopathy.
- Management: Effective management involves addressing the underlying causes and alleviating symptoms:
  - Lifestyle Changes: A low-sodium diet, fluid restriction, and regular physical activity tailored to individual capabilities are essential. Monitoring weight and avoiding excessive fluid intake are also important.
  - Medications: Commonly prescribed medications include diuretics to reduce fluid buildup, ACE inhibitors or ARBs to lower blood pressure, beta-blockers to reduce heart strain, and aldosterone antagonists.
  - Device Therapy: In some cases, devices such as implantable cardioverter-defibrillators (ICDs) or biventricular pacemakers may be used to manage heart failure and improve heart function.

4. Atrial Fibrillation (AFib)

- Overview: AFib is an irregular and often rapid heartbeat that can increase the risk of stroke and other heart-related complications. It is characterized by disorganized electrical signals in the atria.
- Management: Managing AFib involves controlling heart rate, preventing blood clots, and addressing underlying causes:
  - Medications: Antiarrhythmic drugs may be prescribed to control heart rate and rhythm. Anticoagulants, such as warfarin or direct oral anticoagulants (DOACs), help prevent blood clots and reduce the risk of stroke.
  - Procedures: In some cases, procedures such as cardioversion (electrical shock to restore normal rhythm) or catheter ablation (destroying abnormal electrical pathways) may be used to manage AFib.

Medication and Treatment Options

Effective management of heart conditions often requires a combination of medications and treatments tailored to individual needs. Here is an overview of common medications and treatment options:

1. Medications

- Antihypertensives: These include diuretics, ACE inhibitors, ARBs, beta-blockers, and calcium channel blockers. They help lower blood pressure, reduce the risk of complications, and manage symptoms associated with hypertension and heart disease.

- Statins: Statins are used to lower LDL cholesterol levels and reduce the risk of cardiovascular events in individuals with high cholesterol or CAD.

- Antiplatelets and Anticoagulants: Aspirin and other antiplatelet drugs help prevent blood clots, while anticoagulants are used to reduce the risk of clot formation in conditions like AFib or deep vein thrombosis.

- Diuretics: Diuretics help manage fluid retention and reduce symptoms in conditions like heart failure. They work by increasing urine output and reducing fluid buildup in the body.

- Antiarrhythmics: These medications help manage abnormal heart rhythms, including AFib and ventricular arrhythmias. They work by stabilizing electrical activity in the heart.

2. Procedures and Surgical Interventions

- Angioplasty and Stenting: These procedures involve inserting a balloon into narrowed coronary arteries and placing a stent to keep the artery open. They are used to improve blood flow and alleviate symptoms of CAD.

- Coronary Artery Bypass Grafting (CABG): CABG is a surgical procedure that creates a new route for blood to flow around blocked or narrowed coronary arteries. It is used to improve blood supply to the heart muscle and relieve symptoms of CAD.

- Pacemakers and ICDs: Pacemakers are devices that regulate heart rhythm in individuals with abnormal heartbeats. ICDs are used to prevent sudden cardiac death by delivering electrical shocks to correct life-threatening arrhythmias.

- Catheter Ablation: This procedure involves using radiofrequency energy to destroy abnormal electrical pathways in the heart that cause arrhythmias, such as AFib.

Coping Strategies for Chronic Heart Disease

Coping with chronic heart disease involves addressing physical, emotional, and lifestyle challenges to manage symptoms effectively and improve quality of life.

1. Lifestyle Adjustments

- Diet and Nutrition: Adopting a heart-healthy diet is crucial for managing chronic heart conditions. This includes consuming a balanced diet rich in fruits, vegetables, whole grains, lean proteins, and healthy fats. Reducing sodium intake, limiting saturated and trans fats, and avoiding processed foods can help manage blood pressure and cholesterol levels.

- Physical Activity: Regular exercise is beneficial for managing heart disease and improving overall health. Engaging in activities such as walking, swimming, or cycling, tailored to individual capabilities, can help strengthen the heart, improve circulation, and manage weight.

- Stress Management: Chronic stress can exacerbate heart conditions. Incorporating stress-reducing techniques such as mindfulness, relaxation exercises, deep breathing, and engaging in enjoyable activities can help manage stress and improve heart health.

2. Medication Adherence

- Consistency: Adhering to prescribed medications is essential for managing heart conditions effectively. Taking medications as directed by healthcare providers helps control symptoms, prevent complications, and reduce the risk of cardiovascular events.

- Communication: Regular communication with healthcare providers is important for managing medications. Discussing any side effects, concerns, or changes in health status allows for adjustments in treatment plans and ensures optimal management of heart conditions.

3. Support Systems

- Emotional Support: Living with chronic heart disease can be emotionally challenging. Seeking support from family, friends, or support groups can provide encouragement, understanding, and a sense of community.
- Educational Resources: Accessing educational resources about heart disease and management strategies can empower individuals to make informed decisions about their health and actively participate in their care.

4. Regular Monitoring and Follow-Up

- Health Check-Ups: Regular follow-up appointments with healthcare providers are essential for monitoring heart health, assessing treatment effectiveness, and making necessary adjustments. Routine screenings and tests help track progress and identify any potential issues early.
- Self-Monitoring: Monitoring symptoms, blood pressure, weight, and other relevant indicators at home can help individuals stay informed about their health status and detect any changes that may require medical attention.

5. Addressing Coexisting Conditions

- Diabetes Management: For individuals with diabetes, managing blood sugar levels is crucial for heart health. Controlling blood glucose levels can help prevent complications and reduce the risk of cardiovascular disease.

- Mental Health: Addressing mental health issues such as anxiety or depression is important for overall well-being and can positively impact heart health. Seeking professional help and engaging in mental health support can improve quality of life and treatment outcomes.

Creating a Heart-Healthy Lifestyle Plan

Creating a heart-healthy lifestyle plan is essential for maintaining cardiovascular well-being and preventing heart disease. An effective plan involves setting realistic health goals, developing a personalized strategy, and regularly tracking progress while making necessary adjustments. This guide provides a comprehensive approach to creating and implementing a heart-healthy lifestyle plan, addressing each of these key components in detail.

Setting Realistic Health Goals

Setting realistic health goals is the foundation of any successful heart-healthy lifestyle plan. Goals should be specific, measurable, achievable, relevant, and time-bound (SMART). Here's a step-by-step approach to setting and achieving these goals:

1. Identifying Your Health Needs

- Assess Your Current Health Status: Begin by evaluating your current health, including factors such as blood pressure, cholesterol levels, weight, and physical fitness. Understanding your starting point helps in setting informed and realistic goals.
- Consult Healthcare Providers: Seek advice from healthcare professionals to identify specific areas for improvement and receive

personalized recommendations based on your health status and risk factors.

2. Defining SMART Goals

- Specific: Clearly define what you want to achieve. For example, instead of a vague goal like "eat healthier," specify "increase vegetable intake to five servings per day."
- Measurable: Ensure that your goal can be quantified. For instance, "reduce blood pressure by 10 mm Hg" or "lose 10 pounds in three months" are measurable targets.
- Achievable: Set goals that are attainable given your current lifestyle and resources. Avoid setting overly ambitious targets that may lead to frustration.
- Relevant: Align your goals with your overall health objectives. Goals should be pertinent to improving cardiovascular health and addressing personal risk factors.
- Time-Bound: Set a timeline for achieving your goals. A time frame helps create a sense of urgency and facilitates tracking progress. For example, "reduce cholesterol levels within six months."

3. Breaking Down Goals into Actionable Steps

- Create an Action Plan: Divide your main goals into smaller, actionable steps. For example, if your goal is to increase physical

activity, actionable steps might include "start with 15 minutes of daily exercise" and "gradually increase to 30 minutes."
- Prioritize Tasks: Focus on the most important steps first. Prioritizing tasks helps in managing time and resources effectively while maintaining motivation.

4. Building a Support System
- Involve Family and Friends: Share your goals with family and friends who can offer support and encouragement. Their involvement can enhance accountability and provide motivation.
- Seek Professional Help: Consider consulting with a dietitian, fitness trainer, or other specialists who can offer guidance and personalized advice.

Developing a Personalized Heart Health Plan
A personalized heart health plan is tailored to individual needs, preferences, and health conditions. This plan should address key aspects of heart health, including diet, exercise, stress management, and lifestyle modifications.

1. Nutrition and Dietary Changes
- Balanced Diet: Create a meal plan that includes a variety of nutrient-rich foods. Focus on incorporating fruits, vegetables, whole

grains, lean proteins, and healthy fats. Aim for a diet low in saturated fats, trans fats, and cholesterol.

- Portion Control: Practice portion control to manage calorie intake and maintain a healthy weight. Use smaller plates, measure servings, and be mindful of eating habits.

- Hydration: Ensure adequate hydration by drinking plenty of water throughout the day. Limit consumption of sugary beverages and alcohol.

2. Exercise and Physical Activity

- Exercise Routine: Develop a regular exercise routine that includes cardiovascular exercises (e.g., walking, jogging, cycling), strength training (e.g., weight lifting, resistance exercises), and flexibility activities (e.g., stretching, yoga).

- Frequency and Duration: Aim for at least 150 minutes of moderate-intensity aerobic activity or 75 minutes of vigorous-intensity activity per week, along with muscle-strengthening activities on two or more days per week.

- Variety: Incorporate a variety of exercises to keep the routine engaging and address different aspects of fitness. Include activities you enjoy to increase adherence.

3. Stress Management

- Relaxation Techniques: Integrate stress-reducing techniques into your daily routine, such as deep breathing exercises, meditation, or progressive muscle relaxation. These practices can help manage stress and promote overall heart health.
- Mindfulness: Practice mindfulness to stay present and reduce anxiety. Mindfulness techniques can improve emotional well-being and help manage stress effectively.

4. Lifestyle Modifications

- Smoking Cessation: If you smoke, develop a plan to quit. Utilize resources such as nicotine replacement therapy, support groups, or counseling to assist with smoking cessation.
- Alcohol Moderation: Set limits on alcohol consumption to align with recommended guidelines. Opt for lower-alcohol alternatives and engage in activities that do not revolve around drinking.

5. Weight Management

- Healthy Eating: Follow a balanced diet and practice portion control to maintain a healthy weight. Regularly monitor your weight and adjust dietary habits as needed.
- Physical Activity: Incorporate regular physical activity to support weight management and cardiovascular health. Combine aerobic exercise with strength training for optimal results.

Tracking Progress and Making Adjustments

Tracking progress and making adjustments are crucial for maintaining motivation and achieving long-term success in your heart-healthy lifestyle plan. Regularly reviewing your progress helps identify areas of improvement and allows for necessary changes.

1. Monitoring Your Progress

- Set Milestones: Establish short-term and long-term milestones to track progress toward your goals. Celebrate achievements and use them as motivation to continue working toward your objectives.
- Keep Records: Maintain a journal or use a mobile app to track key metrics, such as dietary intake, exercise routines, weight changes, and stress levels. Regularly reviewing these records can provide insights into your progress and areas needing adjustment.
- Evaluate Health Metrics: Regularly monitor health indicators such as blood pressure, cholesterol levels, and weight. Schedule periodic check-ups with healthcare providers to assess overall cardiovascular health.

2. Making Adjustments

- Identify Challenges: Reflect on any obstacles or challenges encountered in achieving your goals. Determine the root causes and develop strategies to address these issues.
- Revise Goals: Adjust your goals as needed based on your progress and changing circumstances. If a goal is no longer relevant or achievable, modify it to better align with your current situation and health objectives.
- Adapt Your Plan: Make necessary changes to your heart health plan based on feedback and progress. For example, if a particular exercise routine becomes monotonous, introduce new activities to maintain engagement and motivation.

3. Seeking Feedback and Support

- Consult Professionals: Seek guidance from healthcare providers, dietitians, or fitness trainers to assess your progress and receive professional input. They can provide valuable recommendations and adjustments to your plan.
- Engage with Support Networks: Continue to involve family, friends, or support groups in your journey. Their encouragement and accountability can help you stay committed to your heart-healthy lifestyle.

4. Maintaining Motivation

- Set New Goals: Once you achieve initial goals, set new, challenging objectives to maintain motivation and continue improving your heart health. For example, if you reach your weight loss target, consider setting a goal for increased physical fitness or improved dietary habits.
- Celebrate Achievements: Acknowledge and reward yourself for reaching milestones. Celebrating your successes can boost morale and reinforce positive behavior.

5. Long-Term Commitment

- Integrate Changes into Daily Life: Ensure that the changes you make become part of your daily routine. Adopting a heart-healthy lifestyle as a long-term commitment helps sustain improvements and prevents relapses.
- Continuous Learning: Stay informed about heart health and wellness through reputable sources. Continuous learning can provide new insights and strategies for maintaining a heart-healthy lifestyle.

Conclusion

In conclusion, maintaining heart health is a dynamic journey that encompasses a range of lifestyle choices and proactive measures. Through this book, we have explored essential strategies for achieving a heart-healthy life, including setting realistic goals, developing a personalized health plan, and incorporating vital lifestyle changes such as nutrition, exercise, stress management, and weight maintenance.

Adopting these practices requires commitment and consistency, but the rewards are profound. By prioritizing heart health, you not only reduce your risk of cardiovascular diseases but also enhance your overall quality of life. Remember, a heart-healthy lifestyle is not a destination but a continuous journey of improvement and well-being.

As you integrate these principles into your daily routine, stay motivated by celebrating your successes and making adjustments as needed. Your dedication to heart health will pave the way for a vibrant, fulfilling life. Embrace these strategies, and take charge of your heart health today for a healthier tomorrow.

www.ingramcontent.com/pod-product-compliance
Lightning Source LLC
Chambersburg PA
CBHW081446250726
48662CB00009B/2962